I0025518

DYNAMICS SHAPING GLOBAL HEALTH SECURITY IN THE NEXT DECADE

NATIONAL INTELLIGENCE ESTIMATE

OFFICE OF THE DIRECTOR OF NATIONAL INTELLIGENCE

NIMBLE BOOKS LLC: THE AI LAB FOR BOOK-LOVERS

~ FRED ZIMMERMAN, EDITOR ~

Humans and AI making books richer, more diverse, and more surprising.

PUBLISHING INFORMATION

(c) 2024 Nimble Books LLC

ISBN: 978-1-60888-254-0

AI-GENERATED KEYWORD PHRASES

Climate change impacts on global health; Direct health effects of climate change; Shifting population demographics and non-communicable diseases; Immunization and TB statistics; Public mistrust and pandemic response; Emerging technological advances in global health.

PUBLISHER'S NOTES

In a world grappling with the long shadow of a still-lethal pandemic and on the brink of unprecedented environmental and social change, understanding the forces shaping our health security is no longer a matter of academic curiosity but one of urgent survival. This book, grounded in rigorous intelligence analysis, offers a roadmap to navigating the complex terrain of global health security, arming you with the knowledge to protect yourself, your loved ones, and your community.

This annotated edition illustrates the capabilities of the AI Lab for Book-Lovers to add context and ease-of-use to manuscripts. It includes several types of abstracts, building from simplest to more complex: TLDR (one word), ELI5, TLDR (vanilla), Scientific Style, and Action Items; essays to increase viewpoint diversity, such as Grounds for Dissent, Red Team Critique, and MAGA Perspective; and Notable Passages and Nutshell Summaries for each page.

ANNOTATIONS

ABSTRACTS

ANALYSIS BASED ON FULL CONTEXT

These analyses are created by using an LLM with a very long input context window, in this case Google Gemini 1.5-pro. The advantage is that the model can use the entirety of the document in its simulated reasoning.

This National Intelligence Estimate (NIE) examines the state of global health security in the aftermath of the COVID-19 pandemic. Climate and societal changes are straining global health resources and increasing the risk of future health emergencies. Health systems, public mistrust and misinformation, and sustained high levels of conflict are impeding national capacities to respond to threats. Adversary interference and uncertainty about the future of the World Health Organization (WHO) are likely to erode global health governance. The report concludes that pandemic fatigue and misinformation may weaken health-seeking behaviors, such as vaccination, and result in significant health emergencies, while donor governments are shifting attention and funding to recent conflicts such as the Israel–Hamas conflict and Russia's war against Ukraine, as well as domestic economic problems. Further straining the international community's ability to address health emergencies, outbreaks of highly pathogenic avian influenza, cholera, dengue, Ebola, monkeypox, and polio have stretched global and national disease detection and response systems.The report assumes that the COVID-19 virus will continue to circulate due to waning immunity following vaccination or infection and naturally evolving viral mutations. However, it also assumes that the virus will continue to cause mostly asymptomatic or mild illness in vaccinated and previously infected individuals, and that combined with improved therapeutics, this will decrease instances of severe disease but will continue to strain already overburdened health systems.

ANALYSIS BASED ON ABRIDGED CONTENT WINDOWS

These analyzes are created by analyzing portions or summaries of the document, using LLMs with shorter context windows. The advantage is that these models are faster and cheaper.

TL;DR (ONE WORD)

Health.

EXPLAIN IT TO ME LIKE I'M FIVE YEARS OLD

In the next ten years, the Earth's climate changing will make people sick and cause big health problems. This is because the weather will get extreme, food will be hard to find, and buildings will break. Also, more people are getting older and living in cities, which will make it hard for doctors and hospitals to help everyone who needs it.

Some diseases like malaria and tuberculosis are still a problem, but there are vaccines and treatments to help. However, some people don't trust the government, which is a problem.

TL;DR (VANILLA)

Climate change and societal changes will strain global health resources and increase the risk of health emergencies in the next decade. Shifting disease patterns, extreme weather, and food insecurity will impact countries worldwide. Changing demographics and the prevalence of non-communicable diseases will strain health systems. Public mistrust and misinformation will undermine response efforts. The use of successful initiatives from the COVID-19 pandemic and emerging technology may help address global health challenges, but some tools may carry unintended risks.

SCIENTIFIC STYLE

This study, approved for public release by the ODNI on 25 April, 2024, presents key judgments on the impact of climate and societal changes on global health resources in the next decade. The analysis indicates a high likelihood of strains on health systems due to increasing climate impacts, such as shifting disease patterns, extreme weather events, food insecurity, and infrastructure destruction. Additionally, changing societal dynamics, including shifting population demographics and a rise in non-communicable diseases, are expected to further stress national and international health systems. The study highlights the importance of building on health advances and emerging technological tools to address global health challenges, while also noting the growing public mistrust and risk of future pandemics.

ACTION ITEMS

Invest in research and development for new technologies and initiatives to address global health challenges, including climate change impacts, shifting demographics, and emerging diseases.

Strengthen international cooperation and coordination to effectively respond to health emergencies and pandemics.

Address public mistrust through transparent and evidence-based communication strategies.

Prioritize investments in healthcare infrastructure and workforce development to meet the growing demands of global health challenges.

Support initiatives to improve access to vaccines and essential healthcare services for vulnerable populations.

Visual Abstracts

Here is a simplified, visually engaging, portrait-oriented color image that conveys the key themes of the "Dynamics Shaping Global Health Security in the Next Decade" without using words or text.

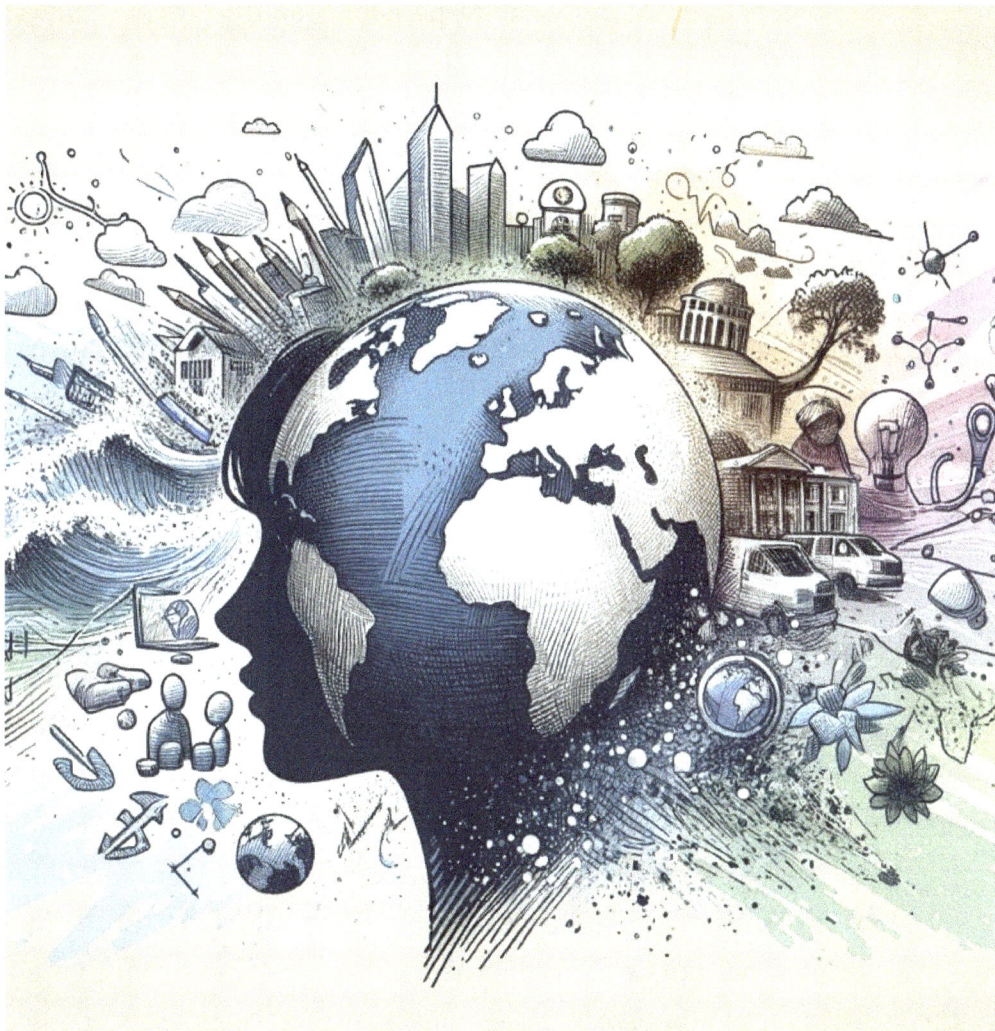

There's a lot going on here. I like the centrality of water, the human mind, urbanization, and youth. —Ed.

VIEWPOINTS

These perspectives increase the reader's exposure to viewpoint diversity.

GROUNDS FOR DISSENT

A member of the organization responsible for this report may have principled, substantive reasons to dissent from the report for several reasons:

Overemphasis on climate change: The member may believe that the report places too much emphasis on the impact of climate change on global health, potentially overlooking other significant factors such as access to healthcare, healthcare infrastructure, and socioeconomic disparities. They may argue that while climate change is certainly a concern, it should not be the sole focus of the report.

Lack of consideration for political factors: The member may believe that the report does not adequately address the role of political factors in shaping global health outcomes. They may argue that political instability, corruption, and conflicts play a significant role in hindering effective health responses, and that these factors should be given more attention in the report.

Skepticism towards technological solutions: The member may be skeptical of the report's optimism towards technological advances as a solution to global health challenges. They may argue that while technology can certainly be helpful, it is not a panacea and may bring unintended consequences or exacerbate existing inequalities in access to healthcare.

Concerns about public distrust: The member may have concerns about the report's focus on growing public mistrust in governments and health sectors. They may argue that this emphasis could lead to a sense of resignation or defeatism, rather than focusing on concrete steps to rebuild trust and improve public health outcomes.

Overall, the member may dissent from the report due to a combination of concerns about its focus, emphasis, and potential blind spots in addressing the complex challenges facing global health in the next decade.

RED TEAM CRITIQUE

Lack of Specificity: The document lacks specificity in terms of the potential impacts of climate change on health and societal dynamics. It makes broad statements about shifting disease patterns, exposure to extreme weather, and food insecurity without providing specific examples or data to support these claims. A more detailed analysis with specific case studies and data would strengthen the credibility of the key judgments.

Lack of Historical Context: The document fails to provide a historical context for the trends it predicts, such as the increasing prevalence of non-communicable diseases and the growing public mistrust in health sectors. Without an analysis of past trends and events, it is difficult to assess the likelihood and severity of the projected impacts.

Limited Focus on Prevention and Mitigation: While the document highlights the potential risks and impacts of climate change and societal changes on global health, it does not emphasize strategies for prevention and mitigation. There is a lack of discussion on proactive measures that can be taken to address these challenges, such as investing in public health infrastructure, promoting sustainable practices, and combating misinformation.

Lack of Alternative Scenarios: The document presents a singular perspective on the potential future of global health, without considering alternative scenarios or potential mitigating factors. A more comprehensive analysis would include a discussion of different possible outcomes and the factors that could influence them, providing a more nuanced and realistic assessment of the situation.

Need for Interdisciplinary Approach: The document would benefit from a more interdisciplinary approach, incorporating insights and perspectives from various fields such as public health, climate science, and social sciences. A more holistic analysis would provide a more well-rounded understanding of the complex interplay between climate change, societal dynamics, and global health.

MAGA Perspective

The so-called "key judgments" presented in this document are nothing but fear-mongering tactics to push a radical climate agenda. The claim that climate change will strain global health resources is a baseless scare tactic meant to control the population and push for more government intervention in our lives. Climate change has been proven to be a natural, cyclical occurrence, and there is no need to panic or drastically alter our way of life.

The mention of shifting population demographics and growing prevalence of non-communicable diseases is simply an attempt to justify more government control over our healthcare systems. The aging population is a natural progression of society, and we should not be using it as an excuse to further infringe on our personal freedoms. Non-communicable diseases are often the result of personal choices and lifestyle habits, and it is not the government's place to intervene in these matters.

The document also mentions public mistrust of governments and health sectors, conveniently leaving out the fact that this mistrust has been fueled by the very institutions that are supposed to protect us. The mishandling of the COVID-19 pandemic and the spread of misinformation by so-called "experts" have eroded public trust in these institutions, and yet they want us to continue to rely on them for our health and safety.

The prediction of a future pandemic is nothing but fear-mongering and an attempt to keep the population in a constant state of alarm. We should not live in fear of hypothetical future events, but rather focus on the present and ensure that our freedoms and rights are protected from government overreach.

Overall, this document is just another tool used by the globalist elite to control the population and push their own agenda. We must resist these tactics and continue to fight for our freedom and sovereignty as a nation.

PAGE-BY-PAGE SUMMARIES

NOTABLE PASSAGES

BODY-2   *During the next decade, the global health security landscape will be shaped by climate and societal changes, strained health infrastructure and capacity, and eroding global health governance. Nonetheless, promising health advances- including the expanded use of successful initiatives developed in response to the COVID-19 pandemic and emerging technological developments- are poised to address some of the shortfalls.*

BODY-3   *During the next decade, the global health security landscape will be stressed by climate and societal changes, strained health infrastructure and capacity, and eroding global health governance. Regardless of the severity and scope, global health emergencies are likely to continue to strain national health systems, particularly disadvantaging poorer countries, as well as encourage and result in responses that are constrained by major power competition. Nonetheless, promising health initiatives utilized during the COVID-19 pandemic, coupled with burgeoning technological advances, are likely to help fill some shortfalls, but will require overcoming competitive approaches and geopolitical rivalry.*

BODY-4   *"We assume that biotechnology advances will continue at the same or increased pace, carrying both opportunities and unintended additional risks. Increasing overlap with other disciplines, including AI, big data analysis, computational simulation techniques, engineering, mathematical modeling, and robotics, are hastening the pace of these advances."*

BODY-5   *During the next decade, climate and societal changes almost certainly will strain global health resources and increase the risk of significant health emergencies. The degree to which national governments prioritize and respond to these concurrent and interconnected risks probably will vary significantly based on perceived immediacy, relative burden, and the ability and willingness to engage with the international community.*

BODY-6   *Climate change is intensifying extreme health events and heat stress, as well as impacting air quality, which will lead to increased fatalities, respiratory and cardiovascular diseases, adverse pregnancy outcomes, mental health effects, and lost worker productivity. The world experienced its hottest summer in recorded human history in 2023, and the UN reported that the world is well off target for necessary emissions reductions, increasing the likelihood of dangerous levels of warming that will impose growing health risks, particularly on lower income countries with less capacity to adapt.*

BODY-7   *Countries worldwide almost certainly will be vulnerable to the direct health effects of climate change, including changing disease patterns or trends, exposure to extreme weather, food insecurity, and infrastructure destruction.*

BODY-8   *"In today's interconnected world, a pathogen can travel from a remote village to a major city in less than 36 hours. In addition to the speed at which the virus that causes COVID-19 spread globally, in 2015, a South Korean visitor to Saudi Arabia acquired Middle East Respiratory Syndrome and spread the disease after returning home, leading to 186 infections, 39 deaths, and $10 billion in damages to the South Korean economy because of containment measures and loss of tourism revenue."*

BODY-9   *"By 2025, the number of people with diabetes worldwide is estimated to more than double to 1.3 billion because of aging populations and surging obesity rates. Separate studies found that by 2045, more than three-quarters of people with diabetes are predicted to live in low- and middle-income countries—owing to* rapidly shifting industrialized lifestyles affecting diet and physical activity—where less than 10 percent of them will have access to diabetes care."

BODY-10   It probably will take years to determine the breadth of the pandemic's impact on these areas.

BODY-11   Many countries are likely to be ill-equipped to manage and contain future health threats because the COVID-19 pandemic accelerated shortages of health care professionals and depleted national health systems, particularly in low- and middle-income countries. Pandemic burnout among health care professionals has amplified staffing shortfalls globally, with a predicted shortage of at least 10 million health care workers by 2030, mostly in low- and middle-income countries. In December 2022, a UN official publicly noted a "very high" incidence of posttraumatic stress disorder in healthcare workers, with many leaving the profession.

BODY-12   The global shortage of healthcare workers is driving an international migration flow of them from low- to high-income countries, with more than 70 countries introducing laws in recent years to facilitate the hiring of foreign health professionals.

BODY-13   "Politically unstable countries, including those recovering from conflict, are at high risk for the emergence of novel pathogens and the reemergence of preventable infectious diseases because of infrastructure and environmental degradation, a scarcity of health care workers, population displacement, and public mistrust fueled by instability and conflict."

BODY-14   "Government disregard for international health norms, adversary interference, and uncertainty about the future of the WHO are likely to erode global health governance during the coming decade. While a lack of government transparency, adversary interference, criticism of national and international public health leadership, struggles to secure the compliance of states with international commitments, and substandard government responses to public health emergencies existed before 2020, the COVID-19 pandemic has renewed attention to these issues."

BODY-15   "Since 2020, China and Russia have used messaging to spread COVID-19 disinformation to undermine trust in Western COVID-19 vaccines, and try to gain greater diplomatic and economic influence. China has remained unwilling to accept foreign COVID-19 vaccine assistance for fear of undermining its narrative that its vaccine was superior and its response to COVID-19 demonstrated superior governance, which left it unprepared to handle a surge of COVID-19 patients when it reversed its zero-COVID policy."

BODY-16   Multiple wars, waning political will, geopolitical rivalries, and low trust among countries increasingly are poised to impede, or even halt, efforts to reach consensus during ongoing negotiations on a pandemic agreement and amendments to the IHRs ahead of the May 2024 deadline.

BODY-17   "The global response to future health crises will hinge on the strength of a pandemic agreement and amendments to the UN's International Health Regulations (IHRs), including the degree to which contentious equity, compliance, and accountability issues are addressed."

BODY-18   "Efforts to improve national health systems could build on the successful implementation of COVID-19 pandemic initiatives—including using technology for disease surveillance and diagnostics, medical delivery, and low-cost programs—to fill health gaps in poorer regions."

BODY-19   *The convergence of biotechnology with other systems—such as AI, cloud computing, materials, and imaging technologies—is enabling new civilian and military applications by accelerating drug discovery, disease surveillance, medical diagnosis, gene editing, and personalized medicine development, although the impact has varied by technology type.*

BODY-20   *"In 2018, a Chinese researcher claimed to have used such a tool to produce HIV-resistant human embryos, purportedly resulting in at least two live births of genetically modified offspring, prompting widespread backlash and projections by some scientists that it would take decades before Western researchers could genetically modify humans at scale."*

BODY-21   *Several emerging technological advances could improve global health, but they also have prohibitive costs, other entry barriers, and potential risks. The biotechnology sector probably requires substantial overhauls of international regulations and standards to address potential weaponization risks and ethical concerns. Increasing overlap with other disciplines, including artificial intelligence, are hastening the pace of advances.*

Approved for Public Release
by ODNI on 25 April, 2024

NATIONAL INTELLIGENCE ESTIMATE

December 2023   NIE 2023-28395-B

Dynamics Shaping Global Health Security In the Next Decade

OFFICE OF THE DIRECTOR OF NATIONAL INTELLIGENCE

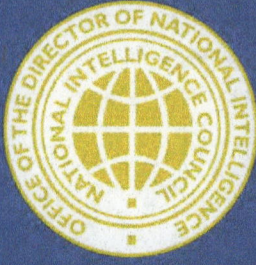

NATIONAL INTELLIGENCE COUNCIL

Approved for Public Release by ODNI on 25 April, 2024

Factors Shaping Global Health Security Through 2033

During the next decade, the global health security landscape will be shaped by climate and societal changes, strained health infrastructure and capacity, and eroding global health governance. Nonetheless, promising health advances—including the expanded use of successful initiatives developed in response to the COVID-19 pandemic and emerging technological developments—are poised to address some of the shortfalls.

CLIMATE AND SOCIETAL FACTORS
- Climate change
- Demographic shifts
- Growing prevalence of non-communicable diseases

INFRASTRUCTURE
- Health system shortfalls
- Public mistrust and medical misinformation
- Strains from conflict

INTERNATIONAL GOVERNANCE
- Disregard for international health institutions and norms
- US adversary interference
- Uncertainty about the future of the WHO

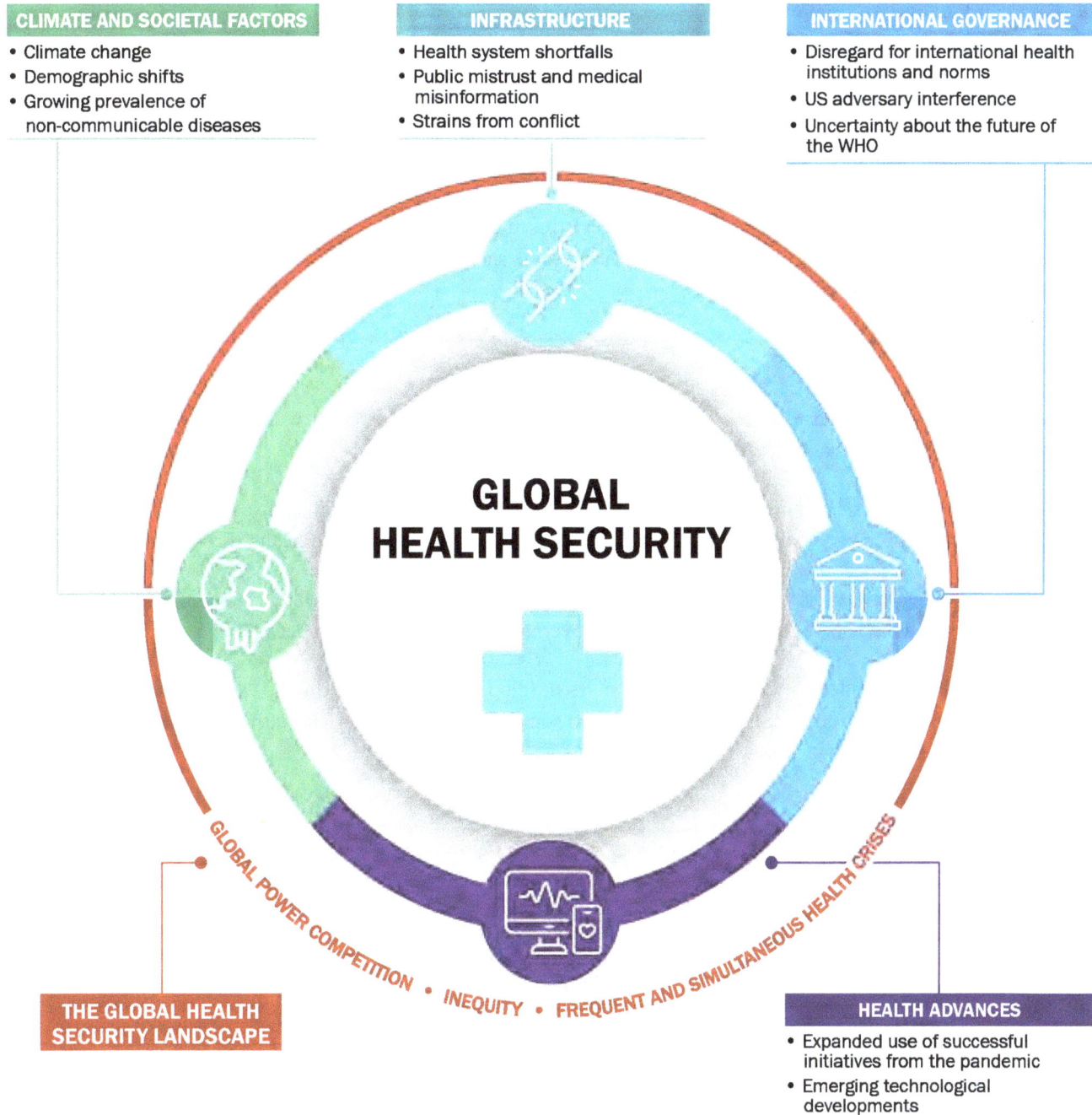

GLOBAL HEALTH SECURITY

GLOBAL POWER COMPETITION • INEQUITY • FREQUENT AND SIMULTANEOUS HEALTH CRISES

THE GLOBAL HEALTH SECURITY LANDSCAPE

HEALTH ADVANCES
- Expanded use of successful initiatives from the pandemic
- Emerging technological developments

2309-01625-A-U2

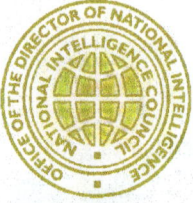

Dynamics Shaping Global Health Security In the Next Decade

December 2023   NIE 2023-28395-B

Key Takeaway

During the next decade, the global health security landscape will be stressed by climate and societal changes, strained health infrastructure and capacity, and eroding global health governance. Regardless of the severity and scope, global health emergencies are likely to continue to strain national health systems, particularly disadvantaging poorer countries, as well as encourage and result in responses that are constrained by major power competition. Nonetheless, promising health initiatives utilized during the COVID-19 pandemic, coupled with burgeoning technological advances, are likely to help fill some shortfalls, but will require overcoming competitive approaches and geopolitical rivalry.

Key Judgment 1: During the next decade, climate and societal changes almost certainly will strain global health resources and increase the risk of significant health emergencies.

Key Judgment 2: Health system shortfalls, public mistrust and medical misinformation, and sustained high levels of conflict and instability are very likely to impede the capacity of countries to respond to health threats through 2033.

Key Judgment 3: Government disregard for international health norms, adversary interference, and uncertainty about the future of the WHO are likely to erode global health governance during the coming decade.

Key Judgment 4: The expanded use of successful initiatives developed in response to the COVID-19 pandemic and emerging technological advances are likely to help address some global health shortfalls, although some tools probably will carry unintended risk.

Scope Note

This National Intelligence Estimate (NIE) examines the state of global health security in the aftermath of the emergency phase of the COVID-19 pandemic. The US Centers for Disease Control and Prevention defines global health security as the existence of strong and resilient public health systems that can prevent, detect, and respond to infectious disease threats. The NIE addresses exogenous factors, national and international health system capacity, and governance issues shaping global health security through 2033, with a focus on the opportunities and risks of burgeoning advances that can fill existing shortfalls. The NIE does not include a discussion about COVID-19 origins or intentional threats from state or non-state actors, such as acts of bioterrorism or use of biological weapons.

Assumptions

We assume that the virus that causes COVID-19 will continue to circulate globally because of waning immunity following vaccination or infection and naturally evolving viral mutations. However, we also assume that the virus will continue to cause mostly asymptomatic or mild illness in vaccinated and previously infected individuals, and that combined with improved therapeutics, this will decrease instances of severe disease but will continue to strain already overburdened health systems.

Despite emerging technological advances that help address some global health shortfalls, we assume that trajectories of long-term drivers such as climate and societal change, global conflict and competition, and humanitarian crises will not be meaningfully altered by health-focused adaptions or response measures in the short term.

We assume that biotechnology advances will continue at the same or increased pace, carrying both opportunities and unintended additional risks. Increasing overlap with other disciplines, including AI, big data analysis, computational simulation techniques, engineering, mathematical modeling, and robotics, are hastening the pace of these advances.

Approved for Public Release by ODNI on 25 April, 2024

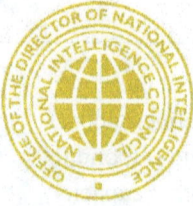

Dynamics Shaping Global Health Security In the Next Decade

December 2023   NIE 2023-28395-B

Discussion

As the international community moves on from the COVID-19 pandemic, strained national and international health systems, pandemic fatigue, contested narratives and misinformation, and competing global priorities, including shifting donor attention and funding, are increasing the risk of backsliding on gains made in health security since 2021. Although not yet fully fulfilled, recent initiatives focused on preparedness, emergency response and funding, and vaccine and therapeutics development and production have advanced previously stalled efforts to improve global health security, including historic negotiations on a pandemic agreement as well as amendments to the UN's International Health Regulations (IHRs). These efforts are at greater risk of stalling, however.

- Pandemic fatigue and medical misinformation may further weaken health-seeking behaviors, such as vaccination, and result in significant health emergencies. Although some child immunization rates have begun to rebound, they still fall short of pre-pandemic coverage particularly in low-income countries.

- Prominent donor governments have shifted their attention and funding from COVID-19 and other global health issues to recent conflicts—such as the Israel–HAMAS conflict and Russia's war against Ukraine—and domestic economic problems. This shift will affect the ability of national health systems to build their pandemic preparedness and address pandemic-related disruptions to more familiar health priorities, such as HIV/AIDS, malaria, maternal and child health, polio, and tuberculosis.

- Further straining the international community's ability to address health emergencies since the height of the pandemic, recent outbreaks of highly pathogenic avian influenza, cholera, dengue, Ebola, monkeypox—now known as mpox—and polio have stretched global and national disease detection and response systems. These crises serve as a reminder of increasingly frequent and simultaneous global health emergencies.

Climate and Societal Dynamics Jeopardizing Global Health

Key Judgment 1: **During the next decade, climate and societal changes almost certainly will strain global health resources and increase the risk of significant health emergencies.** The degree to which national governments prioritize and respond to these concurrent and interconnected risks probably will vary significantly based on perceived immediacy, relative burden, and the ability and willingness to engage with the international community.

Increasing Climate Impacts

Countries worldwide almost certainly will be vulnerable to the increasing direct health effects of climate change, including shifting disease patterns or trends, exposure to extreme weather, food insecurity, and infrastructure destruction. Climate change is undermining global health security by increasing the fragility of socioeconomic systems on which global health depends; expanding the vulnerability of populations to coexisting geopolitical, energy, and cost-of-living increases; and challenging—and potentially reversing—the past 50 years of health gains and widening health inequities between and within populations. The UN estimated that by 2030, the direct annual global health costs of climate change would be between $2 to $4 billion and include additional deaths, the majority of which will occur in

Approved for Public Release by ODNI on 25 April, 2024

Africa and be driven by malaria, malnutrition, diarrhea, and health stress. The World Bank projected that an additional 44 million people would be driven into poverty from health-related climate impacts by 2030 (see figure on page 3).

- Climate-related disease outbreaks are growing because of changes in pathogen characteristics and seasonality and climate hazards that bring people and pathogens closer together; nearly 60 percent of known human pathogenic diseases can be aggravated by climate change. About 4 billion people are currently at risk of contracting mosquito-borne diseases—including dengue and malaria—and researchers expect this number to increase to 4.5 billion by 2050 and 5 billion by 2080 because of climate change.

- Climate change is intensifying extreme health events and heat stress, as well as impacting air quality, which will lead to increased fatalities, respiratory and cardiovascular diseases, adverse pregnancy outcomes, mental health effects, and lost worker productivity. The world experienced its hottest summer in recorded human history in 2023, and the UN reported that the world is well off target for necessary emissions reductions, increasing the likelihood of dangerous levels of warming that will impose growing health risks, particularly on lower income countries with less capacity to adapt. If global mean temperature continues to rise to just under two degrees Celsius, annual heat-related deaths are projected to increase by 370 percent by midcentury, assuming no substantial adaptation progress.

- The UN estimated that by 2050, climate change could increase the risk of food insecurity and malnutrition by 20 percent because of reduced crop yields, poor nutrient quality, and water and sanitation disruptions. Heatwaves alone could lead to nearly 525 million additional people experiencing moderate-to-severe food insecurity by midcentury. One billion children live in the 33 countries that the UN classified as at "extremely high-risk" to the impacts of climate change, with undernutrition accounting for the majority of projected climate-driven child deaths.

- Extreme climate events disrupt health systems, as well as agriculture, electricity, transportation, and water and sanitation networks that affect the provision of health. These disruptions also can impose devastating economic losses—particularly on lower income countries—that can undermine a community's livelihood and ability to afford health care and medicines. In 2022, flooding in Pakistan—affecting more than 33 million people—destroyed 2,000 health facilities, 8,000 kilometers of roads, and the water and sanitation sector in affected areas, which resulted in increased cases of cholera, dengue, malaria, and severe child malnutrition, as well as upticks in maternal and newborn deaths.

Several indirect effects of climate change also will affect global health security. In particular, loss of global biodiversity and potential pathogen spillover from thawing permafrost probably will eliminate potential sources of medical advances and enable disease spread.

- Declining biodiversity—driven by habitat destruction caused by climate and land use changes—is threatening health progress and innovation, food production, and economic prosperity. Such loss jeopardizes global health by facilitating novel disease emergence and eliminating sources for pharmaceutical discovery, including for cancer drugs, antibiotics, antimalarials, and antifungals. Nearly half of all medicines—including 70 percent of cancer drugs—are derived from natural sources.

- Microbes released from melting permafrost by warming temperatures raise the risk of rare, reemerging, or novel pathogen spillovers. In 2016, a child and 2,000 reindeer in Siberia died following exposure to an anthrax-infected reindeer carcass that defrosted during a heatwave; the last outbreak in the region was in 1941.

Approved for Public Release by ODNI on 25 April, 2024

Direct Health Impacts of Climate Change

Countries worldwide almost certainly will be vulnerable to the direct health effects of climate change, including changing disease patterns or trends, exposure to extreme weather, food insecurity, and infrastructure destruction. These effects will have various health impacts and will disproportionately affect individuals living in poorer countries.

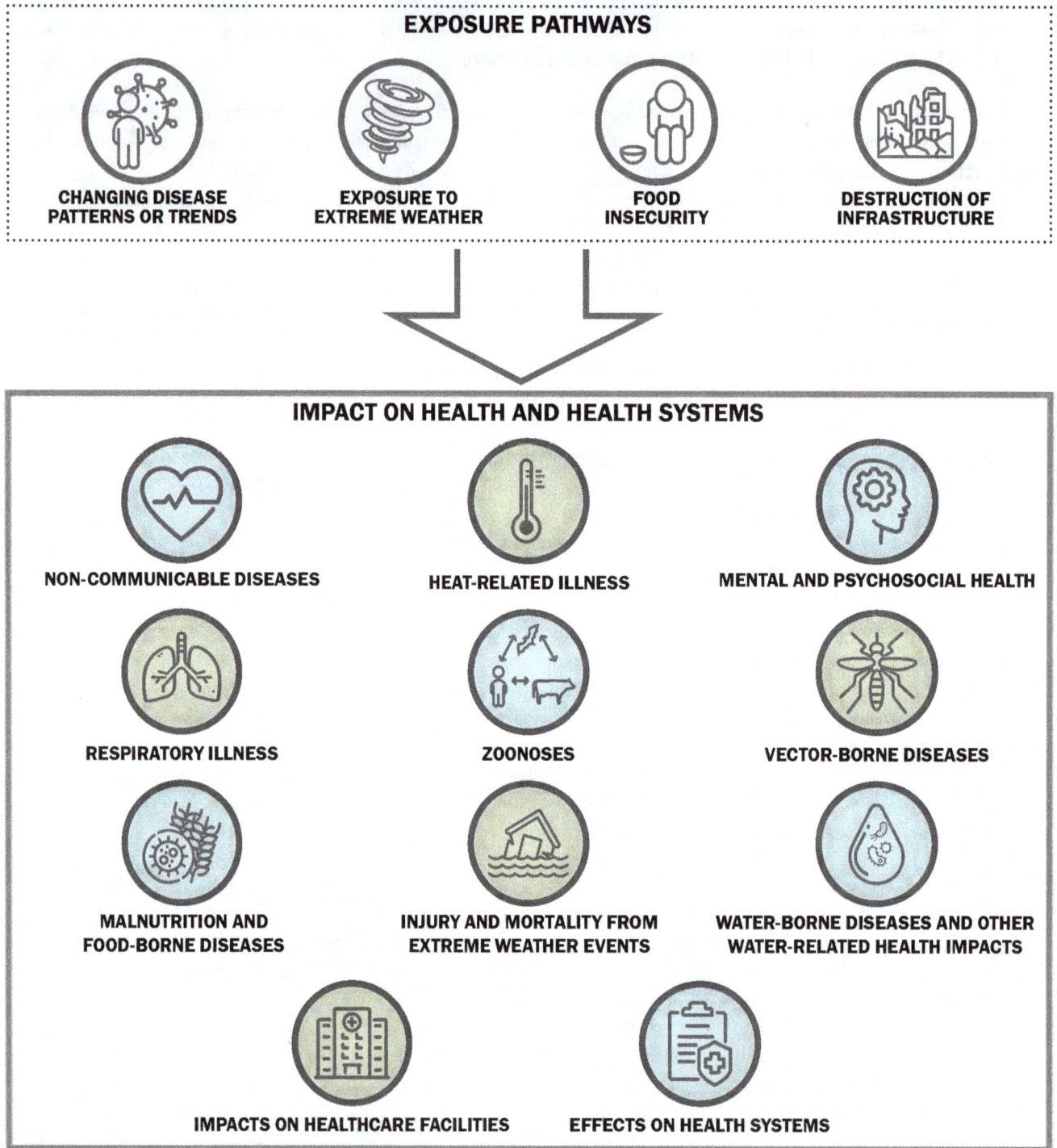

EXPOSURE PATHWAYS

CHANGING DISEASE PATTERNS OR TRENDS — EXPOSURE TO EXTREME WEATHER — FOOD INSECURITY — DESTRUCTION OF INFRASTRUCTURE

IMPACT ON HEALTH AND HEALTH SYSTEMS

NON-COMMUNICABLE DISEASES — HEAT-RELATED ILLNESS — MENTAL AND PSYCHOSOCIAL HEALTH

RESPIRATORY ILLNESS — ZOONOSES — VECTOR-BORNE DISEASES

MALNUTRITION AND FOOD-BORNE DISEASES — INJURY AND MORTALITY FROM EXTREME WEATHER EVENTS — WATER-BORNE DISEASES AND OTHER WATER-RELATED HEALTH IMPACTS

IMPACTS ON HEALTHCARE FACILITIES — EFFECTS ON HEALTH SYSTEMS

2309-01625-B-U2

Approved for Public Release by ODNI on 25 April, 2024

Changing Societal Dynamics

Shifting population demographics—including increased urbanization and rapidly aging populations—and a growing prevalence of non-communicable diseases (NCDs) are likely to significantly strain national and international health systems. During the coming decade, the UN projects that the world's population will increase annually, even as the overall rate of population growth will continue to slow. Expanding populations and increasing internal migration are expected to result in 1.3 billion new urban residents worldwide by 2040, and about 80 percent of this urban growth will happen in poorer regions, including in Sub-Saharan Africa and South Asia.

Outbreaks of infectious diseases, particularly those previously confined to remote areas or in animal populations, are likely to become more frequent because of uncoordinated urbanization, population growth, and expansion of international travel and trade. In addition to the threat of emerging and reemerging diseases, almost 40 percent of urban dwellers currently have no access to safely managed sanitation services, and many lack access to adequate drinking water as well as experience high rates of potentially disabling mental health conditions, such as clinical depression and anxiety disorders.

- The rapid expansion of urban growth into previously uninhabited areas has increased the risk of novel diseases originating in animals spilling over into human populations. Analysis of more than 12,000 infectious disease outbreaks from 1980 to 2013 suggested that the number of outbreaks has increased, in part because pathogens originally found in animals have now spread to human populations. A separate study of novel infectious disease outbreaks during the past 400 years suggests that the annual probability of extreme epidemics occurring could increase threefold in the coming decades.

- Large numbers of unvaccinated people living close to each other in squalid conditions with limited access to primary health care facilities or clean water and sanitation create a fertile breeding ground for infectious disease. In Pakistan, cases of typhoid, which is a result of poor water and sanitation and is vaccine preventable, drastically increased after an unprecedented, extensively drug-resistant outbreak began in the slums of Hyderabad and Karachi in 2016.

- In today's interconnected world, a pathogen can travel from a remote village to a major city in less than 36 hours. In addition to the speed at which the virus that causes COVID-19 spread globally, in 2015, a South Korean visitor to Saudi Arabia acquired Middle East Respiratory Syndrome and spread the disease after returning home, leading to 186 infections, 39 deaths, and $10 billion in damages to the South Korean economy because of containment measures and loss of tourism revenue.

Rapid urbanization and aging populations also will contribute to increasing rates of NCDs—including heart disease, stroke, cancer, diabetes, and chronic lung disease—that are likely to strain the global economy, undermine global health goals, and stress national health systems, particularly in poorer countries. It has been estimated that NCDs will cost the global economy more than $30 trillion between 2011 and 2030, and by 2050, the diseases are projected to account for about 86 percent of global deaths—up from three-quarters currently—because of longer life expectancies, poor nutrition, pollution, and tobacco use.

- In low- and middle-income countries, NCDs often are linked to poverty given they tend to affect people during their most productive years in addition to the strain that high health care expenses and reduced productivity put on developing economies and social and economic development. A study in Nigeria estimated that a household caring for a member with an NCD spent about $400 annually on health care, which is about a quarter of its food expenditure; about 30 percent of these households already were impoverished.

- Increasing rates of NCDs threaten progress toward the UN's Sustainable Development Goals, which seek to end poverty, protect the planet, improve living conditions, and reduce the probability of death from any of the four main NCDs by one-third by 2030. In 2023, the UN reported that small island developing countries in the Caribbean and Pacific regions have the highest prevalence of NCDs and mental health risks, causing a majority of residents to die prematurely. Ten of the island countries have the highest rates of obesity globally, and island countries comprise eight of 15 countries with the highest risk of premature death from cardiovascular disease, cancer, diabetes, or chronic respiratory disease.

- By 2025, the number of people with diabetes worldwide is estimated to more than double to 1.3 billion because of aging populations and surging obesity rates. Separate studies found that by 2045, more than three-quarters of people with diabetes are predicted to live in low- and middle-income countries—owing to rapidly shifting industrialized lifestyles affecting diet and physical activity—where less than 10 percent of them will have access to diabetes care.

Anticipating the Next Pandemic

Although it is impossible to predict when and where the next pandemic will emerge, environments with (1) a high variety of pathogens and frequency of animal disease spillover into humans, (2) a high volume of population movement and trade, and (3) inadequate public health systems and infrastructure are particularly vulnerable. Meeting fewer than all three of these risk factors can still pose a significant risk of large-scale epidemic events, particularly when dynamic socioeconomic and political factors exacerbate exposure and transmission characteristics.

- A novel or emerging respiratory virus, such as influenza or coronavirus, poses the most likely pandemic threat. Respiratory RNA viruses of animal origin are particularly problematic because of difficulty enforcing infection control and containment measures, high mutation rates, and genetic diversity.

Strained Health Infrastructure Impeding Response Capacity

Key Judgment 2: **Health system shortfalls, public mistrust and medical misinformation, and sustained high levels of conflict and instability are very likely to impede the capacity of countries to respond to health threats through 2033.** The COVID-19 pandemic has intensified these challenges and diminished the global health community's ability to detect and respond to the challenge of frequent and simultaneous outbreaks that have the potential to spread worldwide, as well as the ability of key health priorities—such as control methods for HIV/AIDS, malaria, maternal and child health, polio, and tuberculosis—to rebound from disruptions since 2020 (see figure on next page).

Approved for Public Release by ODNI on 25 April, 2024

Global Health Priorities: Status and Future Challenges

Progress in several global health priority areas will be challenged in the coming decade by national health system shortfalls, public mistrust and medical misinformation, and conflict environments. It probably will take years to determine the breadth of the pandemic's impact on these areas.

Stalling   Progressing

Priorities and Progress	Post-Pandemic Realities	Key Challenges in the Coming Decade
Child mortality *(Younger than five years)*	Stagnation in reducing the under-five mortality rate predates the pandemic, which degraded maternal prenatal and postpartum care. COVID-19 infections in children under five years old comprised about 2 percent of global cases and 0.1 percent of deaths. As of 2021, about 5 million children died before reaching their fifth birthday because of preventable or treatable causes; at current rates, about 48 million preventable under-five child deaths will occur by 2030, half of whom will be newborns.	• Lack of prenatal and postpartum care • Insufficient nutrition • Low vaccination rates • Inadequate sanitation and water quality • Poor quality medical care
HIV/AIDS	In 2022, there were about 1.3 million new infections, which is the lowest number since the late 1980s; however, the decline varied by age, sex, race, and region. As of 2022, about 39 million people were living with HIV, up from 31.5 million in 2010, which is the result of continuing infections and people living longer with the disease; about 14 percent of people are unaware they are infected.	• Gender and other inequalities • Violence • Stigma and discrimination • Harmful laws and practices • Funding shortfalls
Immunization	Global immunization services reached 4 million more children in 2022, compared with the previous year; however the number is lower than pre-pandemic levels and disproportionately less in poorer countries. In 2022, about 20.5 million children missed out on one or more vaccines delivered through routine immunization services, compared with 18.4 million children in 2019, representing the largest sustained decline in childhood immunizations in 30 years.	• Pandemic-related disruptions • Anti-vaccine sentiment • Weakened health systems, including health worker shortages and degraded health infrastructure • Public mistrust and misinformation
Malaria	In 2022, the number of malaria cases rose to 249 million, an increase of 5 million cases from the previous year and about 16 million cases more than the pre-pandemic level in 2019. The global malaria incidence was 58.4 cases per 1,000 people, which is off track to meet the WHO target of 26.2 cases by 2025. While the WHO reported that rates of new infections and deaths plateaued in 11 countries with the highest malaria burden, six separate countries were the main sources of the increase in malaria cases.	• Growing global population at risk of contracting the disease • Parasite mutations affecting the performance of rapid diagnostic tests • Growing parasite resistance to anti-malarial drugs • Increasing insecticide resistance • Invasion in Africa of an urban-adapted Asian mosquito • Restricted funding • Climate change

NIC • 2309-01625-C-U2

Approved for Public Release by ODNI on 25 April, 2024

Global Health Priorities: Status and Future Challenges

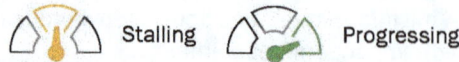

Stalling   Progressing

Priorities and Progress	Post-Pandemic Realities	Key Challenges in the Coming Decade
Maternal mortality	Stagnation in maternal mortality reductions predates the pandemic, which led to COVID-19 infections in pregnant individuals and contributed to pregnancy complications and deaths because of disruptions to health services. Nearly 800 individuals die daily from preventable pregnancy- and childbirth-related causes, and at current rates, about one million preventable maternal deaths will occur by 2030, mostly in low- and middle-income countries.	• Lack of prenatal and postpartum care • Insufficient nutrition • Low vaccination rates • Inadequate sanitation and water quality • Poor quality medical care
Polio	The number of polio cases decreased in 2023 as the Global Polio Eradication Initiative (GPEI) rebounded from the suspension of more than 60 vaccination campaigns during the pandemic. As of late November 2023, the GPEI reported 11 wild polio cases in Afghanistan and Pakistan combined, compared to 140 in 2020. Nonetheless, the goal for ending polio transmission in 2023 will be missed, according to the Independent Monitoring Board of the GPEI.	• Civil unrest • Degraded health infrastructure • Lack of political will
Tuberculosis	In 2022, 7.5 million people were diagnosed with tuberculosis (TB), up from a peak of 7.1 million people in 2019, representing the highest figure recorded since WHO began global TB monitoring in 1995. This number probably includes a backlog of people who developed TB in previous years, but whose diagnosis and treatment were delayed by pandemic-related disruptions. An estimated 10.6 million people were infected with TB in 2022, up from 10.3 million in 2021, however, the number of TB-related deaths was 1.3 million in 2022, down from 1.4 in 2021.	• Conflict-related disruptions to care • Providing and accessing essential TB services for diagnosis and treatment • Declining spending on essential TB services

NIC • 2309-01625-C-U2

Constrained Health System Capacity

Many countries are likely to be ill-equipped to manage and contain future health threats because the COVID-19 pandemic accelerated shortages of health care professionals and depleted national health systems, particularly in low- and middle-income countries. Pandemic burnout among health care professionals has amplified staffing shortfalls globally, with a predicted shortage of at least 10 million health care workers by 2030, mostly in low- and middle-income countries. In December 2022, a UN official publicly noted a "very high" incidence of posttraumatic stress disorder in healthcare workers, with many leaving the profession.

- In October 2022, pandemic-related shortages of healthcare workers, COVID-19 burnout, and poor capacity for disease detection left Uganda's private clinics without enough trained clinicians and adequate safety precautions to respond to an Ebola outbreak. The shortfalls prolonged the outbreak by impeding accurate diagnosis, disease containment, and efforts to prevent deaths of health care professionals.

Approved for Public Release by ODNI on 25 April, 2024

- In 2022, Malawi's health system was overburdened as it attempted to address its first polio outbreak in 30 years—tied to a strain that circulated in Pakistan in late 2019—and an unusually persistent cholera outbreak. A health official attributed the polio outbreak to Malawi's depleted health system—the initial patient was not fully immunized—and gaps in global surveillance after the emergency phase of the pandemic.

- The global shortage of healthcare workers is driving an international migration flow of them from low- to high-income countries, with more than 70 countries introducing laws in recent years to facilitate the hiring of foreign health professionals.

- Overburdened health care systems and shortfalls in sanitation, disease diagnostics, and prudent use and regulation of antibiotics have contributed to a rise in antimicrobial resistance (AMR). Low-income countries are particularly vulnerable to AMR and its spread because infectious diseases are more common, health systems are weaker, and the economic burden is greater, as less expensive first-line antibiotics become less effective. The UN estimated that by 2050, AMR would cause 10 million deaths, up from 1.27 million in 2022. The UN also projected that AMR would cause global GDP to decrease by at least $3.4 trillion annually by the end of the decade, pushing some 24 million people into extreme poverty because of high treatment costs and illness-related wage loses.

Growing Public Mistrust

The uneven public health response to the COVID-19 pandemic and medical misinformation have stoked sustained public distrust of governments and health sectors that almost certainly will undermine response efforts for other diseases during the next decade. Increased adoption of communications technologies, more permissive information environments, and the political aspects of this particular pandemic that provided a fertile setting for myriad social and technological forces to breed confusion and distrust have all furthered the growth of medical misinformation, which is likely to persist during the next several years. This environment also has cultivated state-sponsored disinformation, which has purposefully contributed to public mistrust.

- Globally, the health response to the pandemic has undermined public trust in governments, which fell in 14 of 26 countries surveyed last year. Many publics worldwide viewed governmental pandemic responses as poorly communicated and impinging on personal sovereignty, according to an independent report by the WHO; in December 2022, global health officials noted that misinformation and vaccine hesitancy were at all-time highs, with people less motivated to follow recommended protective health behaviors for COVID-19 and other health threats.

- In January 2023, some Malawian communities—rife with pandemic conspiracy theories—chased away healthcare professionals who were administering the cholera vaccine and accused them of trying to trick people into taking the COVID-19 vaccine. Tanzania reported that the misinformation about COVID-19 vaccines reduced public confidence in vaccines and contributed to a decline in childhood immunization rates in 2021.

- In 2022, pockets of mpox misinformation and vaccine hesitancy—some of which stemmed from inaccuracies in COVID-19 vaccine information—almost certainly slowed containment efforts in several countries.

- In 2022, public mistrust of Uganda's Ebola response inhibited detection and containment by fueling misconceptions about the disease. Patients fled isolation or sought care beyond Ebola treatment centers.

- Health controversies and medical misinformation of these kinds can amplify disease transmission and have costly and disruptive effects. Although a study in 1998 in a UK medical journal that linked autism and bowel disorders with the combined measles, mumps, and rubella vaccine has been retracted, it heightened concerns worldwide—still lingering today—and has been associated with anti-vaccine sentiment and increases in measles outbreaks originating in unimmunized populations.

Record Conflicts and Crises

Record levels of conflict, instability, and prolonged humanitarian crises in the world that also are more protracted than in recent decades are likely to lead to large-scale population displacements and associated negative health effects, including increasing disease transmission. Conflicts are now lasting more than 20 years on average, an increase from about 13 years in the mid-1980s, and as of June 2023, 360 million people were in need of humanitarian assistance, an increase of 30 percent since early 2022.

- Politically unstable countries, including those recovering from conflict, are at high risk for the emergence of novel pathogens and the reemergence of preventable infectious diseases because of infrastructure and environmental degradation, a scarcity of health care workers, population displacement, and public mistrust fueled by instability and conflict. Trends in increased violence worldwide during the next two decades could reverse global health security progress, with the WHO estimating that 80 percent of major disease outbreaks are occurring in fragile and vulnerable countries.

- A coalition of international NGOs reported nearly 2,000 attacks against health care facilities and personnel in 2022, an increase of 45 percent since the previous year and the highest number in at least a decade. The report cited an increasing number of attacks against vaccination campaigns, particularly in Afghanistan, Burma, Mali, Nigeria, Pakistan, South Sudan, and Sudan.

- The WHO has reported record outbreaks of preventable diseases in conflict-ridden countries, including the world's largest cholera outbreak in Yemen, the world's second-largest Ebola outbreak in eastern Democratic Republic of the Congo, and unprecedented outbreaks of diphtheria, malaria, measles, and tuberculosis in Venezuela.

Uneven Biosafety Practices Increase Risk of Disease Outbreaks

The proliferation of high-containment biological laboratories and highly technical molecular laboratory capabilities, coupled with minimal expert oversight and an uneven and decentralized biosafety regulatory environment, probably has increased the risk of pathogen containment exposures and subsequent outbreak of disease. Since 2000, the number of biosafety level-4 (BSL-4) and BSL-3 laboratories, which handle the most deadly disease agents, has significantly increased. Since the COVID-19 pandemic, a growing number of laboratories have received molecular testing capabilities and platforms for disease diagnostics and infectious disease research, but this often is conducted at lower containment levels than recommended by the WHO, putting the total number of facilities handling dangerous pathogens in the tens of thousands.

- Countries are responsible for establishing and enforcing their own biosafety requirements, resulting in vast disparities in biosafety features. BSL-3 and BSL-4 laboratories increasingly do not meet biosafety guidelines set by the WHO, partly because of a lack of international inspections and registration requirements, and in some instances, because unsafe biosafety practices involve work being conducted at a lower biosafety level than recommended for a pathogen.

- Poor biosafety practices have led to previous disease outbreaks, including a single case of Ebola in Russia and localized cases of Severe Acute Respiratory Syndrome (SARS) in Taiwan, according to the WHO and the

NIC ▐▌▌▐▌▌▐▌▌▐▌   NATIONAL INTELLIGENCE COUNCIL

US Centers for Disease Control and Prevention. In addition, the 1977-78 H1N1 influenza pandemic that led to the reemergence of an older and noncirculating strain probably was the result of a laboratory-acquired infection or laboratory accident in Russia, according to scientific journal articles and international press reports.

Lack of Transparency, Global Competition, Uncertainty About WHO Eroding Global Health Governance

Key Judgment 3: **Government disregard for international health norms, adversary interference, and uncertainty about the future of the WHO are likely to erode global health governance during the coming decade.** While a lack of government transparency, adversary interference, criticism of national and international public health leadership, struggles to secure the compliance of states with international commitments, and substandard government responses to public health emergencies existed before 2020, the COVID-19 pandemic has renewed attention to these issues.

Lack of Government Transparency

Since the pandemic, a lack of transparency by governments and organizations related to health developments almost certainly will undermine public trust and weaken adherence to the UN's health protocols, increasing the risk of widespread disease transmission. This opacity—driven in part by authorities wanting to avert criticism, avoid economic damage, or appear in control—coincides with high global attention on how to improve national and international outbreak response efforts in the aftermath of the pandemic.

- In April 2023, the WHO reported that China's National Health Commission provided notification of a confirmed human H3N8 avian influenza infection—the third reported human case and first death—24 days after the patient was hospitalized and 11 days after the patient died. The UN's IHRs—requirements for countries to respond to and contain significant health threats—obligate countries to report human infections with nonhuman influenza strains immediately.

- The Equatoguinean Government's lagging communication about a Marburg outbreak in 2023 drove disease spread and prolonged the health crisis.

- In March 2023, many African and international leaders expressed concern about the AU's appointment of a new director general of the Africa Centers for Disease Control and Prevention (CDC), claiming the selection process was "excessively secretive." This is likely to weaken the Africa CDC's credibility with the international community and African member states as it seeks to transition from a specialized technical institute of the AU into a public health agency with more authority, speed, and flexibility in responding to health crises.

Adversary Interference

During the coming decade, adversaries probably will impede efforts to reach consensus in key ongoing global health negotiations and forums as part of their efforts to compete with the United States for influence, which may undermine the broader global health governance architecture and key cooperative initiatives. These include WHO member state efforts aimed at strengthening global preparedness and response to health crises through ongoing negotiations on a pandemic agreement and amendments to the IHRs or other high-level UN initiatives (see figure on page 13). In September 2023, ahead of several UN General Assembly high-level meetings on health topics, Belarus, Bolivia, Cuba, Eritrea, Iran, Nicaragua, North Korea, Russia, Syria, Venezuela, and Zimbabwe threatened to block the adoption of

Approved for Public Release by ODNI on 25 April, 2024

political declarations on pandemic preparedness and response, universal health coverage, tuberculosis, and the UN's Sustainable Development Goals.

- Russia is trying to subvert longstanding norms of WHO governance and consensus-making. In May 2023, Russia forced the first vote since 1977 on membership to the WHO's Executive Board to contest Ukraine's nomination by the European region after member states condemned Russian attacks on Ukrainian health facilities and pushed the WHO to close a noncommunicable disease office in Moscow.

- Russia is working with several other countries to weaken or block language on LGBTQIA+ and gender issues on several health items.

- In May 2023, North Korea secured, through the WHO South East Asia region, a three-year position on the WHO's Executive Board, which informs the decisions and policies of the World Health Assembly (WHA), the governance body of the WHO. Pyongyang often has resisted collaborating with international organizations, including the WHO, on health issues, such as a COVID-19 outbreak last year.

- China has actively spoken up in support of African countries in pandemic agreement negotiations on equity topics in opposition to US positions, such as on intellectual property rights and technology transfers. China also is a strong participant in the Group for Equity in pandemic agreement negotiations, representing 20 member states, largely from the Global South.

- Since 2020, China and Russia have used messaging to spread COVID-19 disinformation to undermine trust in Western COVID-19 vaccines, and try to gain greater diplomatic and economic influence. China has remained unwilling to accept foreign COVID-19 vaccine assistance for fear of undermining its narrative that its vaccine was superior and its response to COVID-19 demonstrated superior governance, which left it unprepared to handle a surge of COVID-19 patients when it reversed its zero-COVID policy. More recently, for instance, Russian actors have promoted disinformation throughout the global mpox outbreak to denigrate the United States and stoke societal tension in the West, according to Russian state media.

Delays in WHO Reforms

The success of the international community's efforts to strengthen the WHO's independence, authority, reliable funding, and efficient processes by 2024 almost certainly will shape the trajectory of global health governance, but this is highly uncertain because of the geopolitical competition that threatens to impede collective approaches to health security. Health experts and WHO member states, although critical of the WHO's slow response during the COVID-19 pandemic, have acknowledged the unique role the organization plays in managing global health emergencies.

- The IHRs govern global responses to international public health threats, and WHO member states will continue to discuss amendments to give the WHO freedom to communicate on disease outbreaks, declare a public health emergency based on scientific considerations, and investigate without hindrance. WHO member states will continue to negotiate adjustments, with the goal of approving amendments in May 2024, although changes probably will take years to implement.

- In January 2023, the WHO stated that a pandemic agreement would reinforce its legitimacy and authority. WHO member states continue to negotiate a draft of a pandemic agreement, aimed at preventing global disease outbreaks and better coordinating a worldwide response, with the final draft due to the WHA in May 2024.

- In May 2023, WHO member states adopted a 20-percent increase in assessed contributions contingent on ongoing WHO reform measures. The action signified a tangible commitment to increase assessed contributions

Approved for Public Release by ODNI on 25 April, 2024

NIC ‖‖‖‖‖‖‖ NATIONAL INTELLIGENCE COUNCIL

by as much as 50 percent by 2030, a recommendation adopted in 2022. The WHO's budget has long comprised voluntary contributions earmarked for specific programs, restricting the WHO's flexibility to respond to ad hoc needs.

- In late 2022, WHO Director General Tedros Adhanom noted that he had worked to increase efficiency by decreasing the number of WHO assistant director generals, downgrading several senior positions, and flattening the organizational structure of some entities, including the WHO's Health Emergency team. Tedros will stay in his position until mid-2027, at which time a new director general will be elected.

- Multiple wars, waning political will, geopolitical rivalries, and low trust among countries increasingly are poised to impede, or even halt, efforts to reach consensus during ongoing negotiations on a pandemic agreement and amendments to the IHRs ahead of the May 2024 deadline.

Wildcards That Could Alter our Analysis

Two wildcards that could quickly alter the global health landscape during the coming decade include another pandemic or a significant shift in political will and funding for global health security.

- **Pandemic.** A pandemic that is similar or worse than COVID-19 during the next 10 years would significantly challenge the ability of countries and the international community to respond, causing a range of global economic, human security, governance, and geopolitical strains. A study of novel infectious disease outbreaks in the past 400 years suggested that the probability of a pandemic with impact similar to that of COVID-19 is about 2 percent annually, with the probability of experiencing one during one's lifetime at about 38 percent. A separate study projected a nearly 28 percent chance that a pandemic at least as deadly as COVID-19 would occur during the next decade.

- **Political Will and Funding.** A substantial increase or decrease in high-level attention and funding for global health security—because of a significant world event or health crisis—almost certainly would shift the global prioritization of health security. International funding for global health security typically increases during a significant disease outbreak and decreases after the emergency has subsided, resulting in a cycle of panic and neglect. This pattern occurred with the Severe Acute Respiratory Syndrome (SARS) outbreak during 2002-04, the H1N1 influenza pandemic in 2009, the Ebola outbreak in West Africa during 2014-16, and the COVID-19 pandemic.

Approved for Public Release by ODNI on 25 April, 2024

Future Global Health Responses Hinge on Equity, Accountability, and Compliance

The global response to future health crises will hinge on the strength of a pandemic agreement and amendments to the UN's International Health Regulations (IHRs), including the degree to which contentious equity, compliance, and accountability issues are addressed. Member states and blocs have held fast to their positions on equity and national sovereignty issues in ongoing negotiations. This issue predates the pandemic, with countries failing to promptly report dangerous disease outbreaks, share pathogen and genomic sequence data, and equitably distribute lifesaving vaccines and therapeutics.

EQUITY

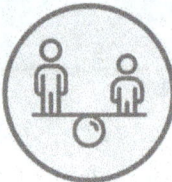

Developed and developing countries were increasingly at odds during pandemic agreement discussions as countries differ sharply on how to address sensitive equity issues, such as intellectual property, technology access, and benefit sharing. High-income countries prioritize full access to scientific data, such as pathogen and genomic sequencing data, but lower-income countries want assurances that if data are shared, they will have access to lifesaving vaccines and drugs.

ACCOUNTABILITY

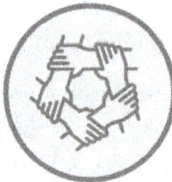

Some member states believe that increased accountability, such as an independent oversight mechanism empowered to investigate outbreaks or potential violations in transparency, would impinge on a country's independence. Some countries have demanded that any efforts that broaden the WHO's authority in outbreaks and emergency response must be based on national sovereignty and consent. Allegations that the WHO is trying to use the pandemic accord to grow its power at the expense of national sovereignty has proliferated around the world.

COMPLIANCE

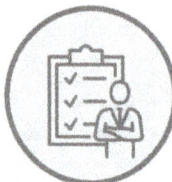

Without effective mechanisms, countries will not abide by their international obligations, including transparency in timely reporting of disease outbreaks, judging from past noncompliance to the IHRs.

NIC • 2309-01625-D-U2

Approved for Public Release by ODNI on 25 April, 2024

Building on Health Advances and Burgeoning Technology

Key Judgment 4: **The expanded use of successful initiatives developed in response to the COVID-19 pandemic and emerging technological advances are likely to help address some global health shortfalls, although some tools probably will carry unintended risk.** Many health issues do not require a technological solution, making biotechnology gains less applicable. As with the potential for the WHO to play a stronger role, however, maximum benefits from the acceptance and application of lessons learned and key initiatives developed in response to COVID-19 as well as new technologies will require overcoming competitive approaches and geopolitical rivalry among leading world powers.

Expanding on Nascent Gains

Efforts to improve national health systems could build on the successful implementation of COVID-19 pandemic initiatives—including using technology for disease surveillance and diagnostics, medical delivery, and low-cost programs—to fill health gaps in poorer regions. Expanded use of these tools by regional and national entities in underserved areas could mitigate the strain on health care systems in countries such as India where 20 percent of the country's hospitals care for more than 60 percent of the population.

- Wastewater surveillance technologies advanced rapidly during the pandemic, offering a potentially more efficient, health care-independent, and timely means to detect disease outbreaks than existing techniques. More than 55 countries have used advanced wastewater surveillance techniques to identify COVID-19 surges, with the potential to expand deployment to low-income countries to monitor for diseases such as poliovirus, rotavirus, or cholera.

- The pandemic advanced efforts to use UAVs to deliver medical supplies and since at least 2019, Ghana, India, Japan, Kenya, Malawi, Nigeria, Russia, Rwanda, Uganda, and the UAE have pursued UAVs to facilitate the rapid delivery of medical supplies to remote areas. The Malawian Government and the UN have used drones to deliver essential medical supplies to 60 remote facilities across six districts in the country, including providing essential immunizations to inaccessible areas following Cyclone Freddy. During the past decade in Rwanda, drones have served nearly 4,000 health facilities, made 13 million vaccine deliveries, and are responsible for transporting 75 percent of the country's national blood supply outside Kigali.

- Physical distancing and the need for rapid data collection during the pandemic have led more low-income countries to adopt telemedicine—relaying medical advice by telephone or online means—and electronic health techniques, such as virtual consultations. In 2020, the WHO reported that nearly 60 percent of countries worldwide were using telemedicine measures to replace in-person consultations, providing a means to serve high-risk individuals and boost efforts in low-income countries; less than 40 percent of low-income countries reported using such measures before the pandemic.

- A public health expert suggested that the pandemic has accelerated health policy changes to simplify the delivery of care, such as shifting basic services from physicians to community health workers, distributing some prescription drugs over the counter, and providing multimonth distributions of antiretroviral therapies for HIV/AIDS and tuberculosis treatment. Rwandan health officials have piloted the use of robots to deliver food, drugs, and other necessities to quarantined patients with COVID-19, reducing health care workers' exposure to the disease.

Approved for Public Release by ODNI on 25 April, 2024

The implementation of these nascent gains will hinge on strengthening public-private partnerships to share the technologies and platforms, as well as increasing the role of international and local NGOs to train public health officials and health care workers in the new initiatives. Sustained diplomatic engagement and international financing almost certainly will be required to spur governments and donors to make sufficient investments in these initiatives to strengthen their national health systems. However, international funding for global health security, which goes primarily to developing countries, typically increases during a significant disease outbreak and decreases after the emergency has subsided.

Global Climate Mitigation and Adaptation Measures Offer Multiple Health Benefits

International actions to mitigate climate change through reducing global greenhouse gas emissions and helping societies adapt to increasing climate impacts also present multiple health benefits. Global efforts to reduce greenhouse gas emissions, if accelerated, would slow the trajectory of climate change, limit the scope and intensity of future extreme weather events, and avert the most catastrophic effects.

- Reducing global fossil fuel usage would offer notable health co-benefits, including helping to lower the number of people, currently 1.2 million, who die annually because of particulate matter (PM 2.5) pollution. Efforts by governments to adapt their societies to climate change by investing in drought-resistant crops, extreme weather early warning systems, and specialized disease surveillance tools, also would help lessen the health-related risks of climate change.

Emerging Technological Advances

Several emerging technological advances—including but not limited to the integration of AI with biotechnology, synthetic biology, precision medicine, and genomics—could improve global health, but also carry risk or prohibitive costs, which may constrain use in low-resource environments and exacerbate existing disparities (see figure on page 17).

- The convergence of biotechnology with other systems—such as AI, cloud computing, materials, and imaging technologies—is enabling new civilian and military applications by accelerating drug discovery, disease surveillance, medical diagnosis, gene editing, and personalized medicine development, although the impact has varied by technology type. During the pandemic, several countries used AI technologies to track COVID-19 infections and vaccinations, provide early case detection, connect patients with medical resources, and enforce mask wearing.

- Advances in synthetic biology—the field of designing and manufacturing biological parts, systems, and organisms—are poised to transform crop and livestock agriculture, building materials, chemical production, environmental mitigation, and health care potentially in ways not seen since the Industrial Revolution. Scientists are building on biomanufacturing, which uses biological systems to improve existing products and develop new ones, to design and build new drugs, vaccines, and cell therapies that can treat and cure diseases, although current infrastructure is limited.

- Health care probably will increasingly include highly personalized medications, therapeutics, and treatments based on genetics, medical history, health behaviors, and lifestyle with an emphasis on improving patient outcomes, particularly in wealthy countries that can afford to develop and implement these approaches. For instance, some researchers are developing vaccines that specifically target the cancer cells of individuals' tumors to help their immune systems recognize and destroy those cells.

- Advances in the accuracy and efficiency of gene editing and DNA synthesis tools could enhance public health capabilities, but these approaches present a range of ethical and geopolitical dilemmas. Since 2017, researchers have refined CRISPR-based systems to enable rapid detection of pathogens and distinguish between closely related strains of viruses or bacteria. Researchers also have used synthetic biology and DNA synthesis techniques to show that viruses could be constructed or recreated in a laboratory, allowing novel viruses to be studied for biomedical or pharmaceutical purposes. In 2018, a Chinese researcher claimed to have used such a tool to produce HIV-resistant human embryos, purportedly resulting in at least two live births of genetically modified offspring, prompting widespread backlash and projections by some scientists that it would take decades before Western researchers could genetically modify humans at scale.

- The diagnosis, treatment, or even elimination of many common diseases may become more feasible, spurred on by a range of biotechnology advances, including vector control,[a] CRISPR-based technologies that have made it easier to modify organisms' genomes, and the development of new medical treatments and preventative medicines. Since 2015, Western researchers have sought to use CRISPR-based gene drives in mosquitoes to reduce or eliminate mosquito-borne diseases such as malaria and the Zika virus, and have successfully developed gene drive-harboring mice. These advances risk unintended consequences of organisms interacting or responding in unexpected ways, proving difficult to control or unpredictably disrupting ecosystems, although such developments are subject to oversight and scrutiny to minimize environmental impacts.

The biotechnology sector has far-reaching potential, but also probably requires substantial overhauls of international regulations and standards to address weaponization risks and ethical concerns, as well as the implementation of security protocols to safeguard critical health information and pharmaceutical infrastructure. Certain subsectors also probably require a sustained increase in scientific knowledge and biomanufacturing infrastructure to reach their promise and will continue to face barriers to implementation, including start-up funding, the time to secure approval and commercialization, and talent. Biotechnology advances also can encourage geopolitical competition, which can result in a race for supremacy to produce products of better quality or in a more timely fashion, as well as ethical challenges and inequities, particularly if adoption is uneven worldwide.

---

[a] Vector control aims to limit the transmission of pathogens by reducing or eliminating human contact with the vector.

Technology Advances in Global Health: Barriers and Risks

Several emerging technological advances could improve global health, but they also have prohibitive costs, other entry barriers, and potential risks. The biotechnology sector probably requires substantial overhauls of international regulations and standards to address potential weaponization risks and ethical concerns. Increasing overlap with other disciplines, including artificial intelligence, are hastening the pace of advances.

The degree of maturity varies by sector, with some advances, such as disease surveillance, being mature, and others, such as disease eradication, being less mature.

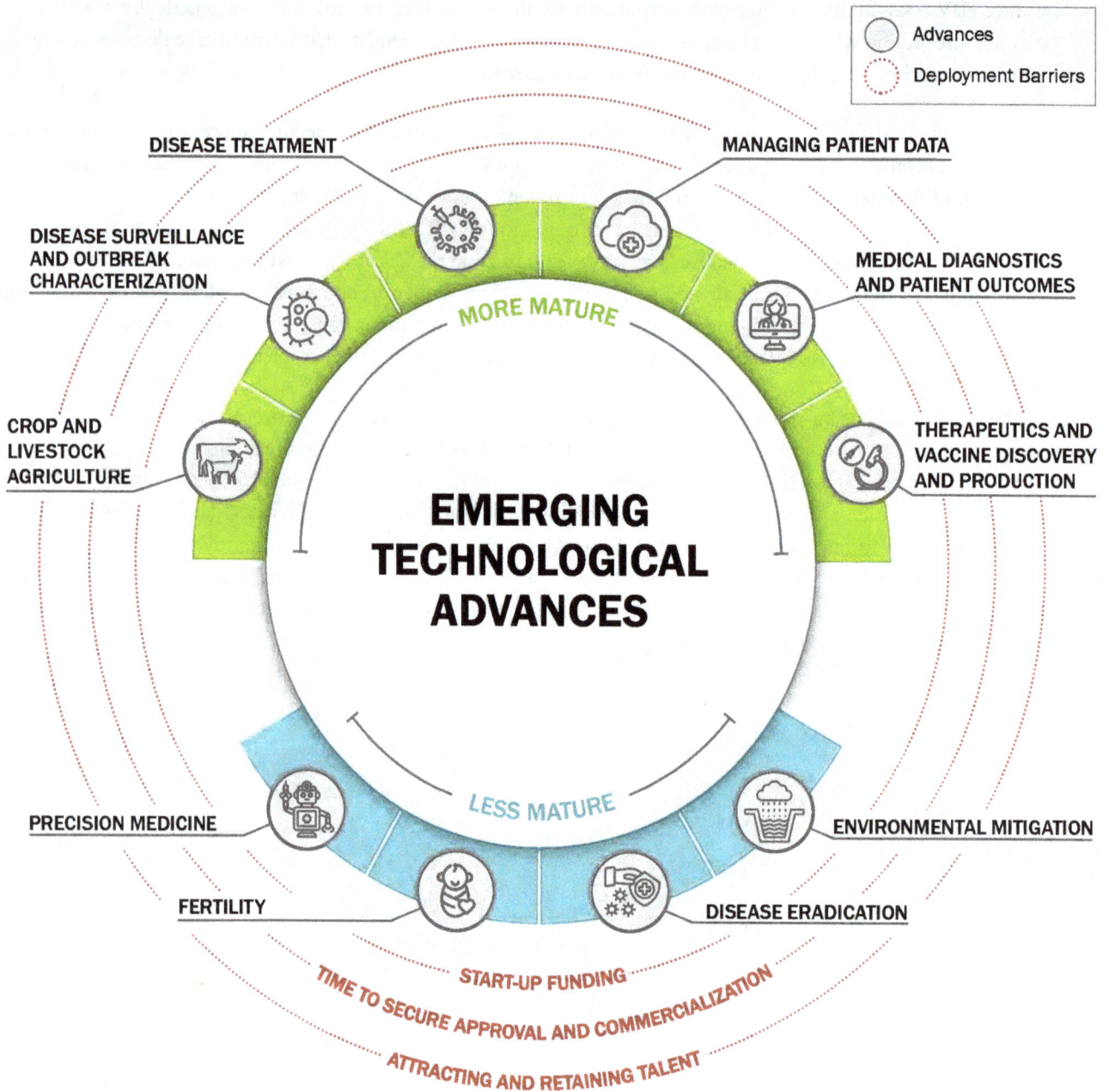

Advances

Deployment Barriers

DISEASE TREATMENT

MANAGING PATIENT DATA

DISEASE SURVEILLANCE AND OUTBREAK CHARACTERIZATION

MEDICAL DIAGNOSTICS AND PATIENT OUTCOMES

MORE MATURE

CROP AND LIVESTOCK AGRICULTURE

THERAPEUTICS AND VACCINE DISCOVERY AND PRODUCTION

EMERGING TECHNOLOGICAL ADVANCES

PRECISION MEDICINE

ENVIRONMENTAL MITIGATION

LESS MATURE

FERTILITY

DISEASE ERADICATION

START-UP FUNDING

TIME TO SECURE APPROVAL AND COMMERCIALIZATION

ATTRACTING AND RETAINING TALENT

NIC • 2309-01625-E-U2

www.ingramcontent.com/pod-product-compliance
Lightning Source LLC
Chambersburg PA
CBHW080058280326
41934CB00014B/3356